Keto diet for beginners

Contents

A ketogenic diet is a low-carb, medium-protein, and high-fat diet that turns the body **into a fat burning machine**.

Several studies and researches have seen that this diet has many health benefits for the body and mind and treatment of some diseases in addition to its effectiveness in losing weight effectively.

What distinguishes the keto diet or low-carb diet is that a person does not feel hungry and does not count calories heavily when following a keto diet or low-carb diet in general.

In this detailed book, you'll find all the information you need in detail to properly follow the keto diet, let's start

What is the keto diet?

Keto is a diet used in the early 1900s to treat epilepsy in children. Later, scientists noticed the effect of this system on losing weight very effectively and quickly.

Keto is a diet that powers the body through fat rather than carbohydrates. Where the nutritional values are: 70-80% fats, 20-25 proteins, 5-10 carbohydrates, most fats are from the body's need for calories instead of carbohydrates.

The ketogenic diet is derived from the name Keto. They are small fuel molecules called ketones.

These molecules are stored in the liver as an alternative energy source. When there is no primary source of energy, glucose and insulin, these molecules are burned as an alternative energy source.

Ketones are produced when you eat a small amount of carbohydrates. These molecules are distributed and analyzed in blood sugar, and the additional protein is converted to blood sugar.

These ketones are produced and stored in the liver from fat sources, and then used as fuel throughout the body, including the brain.

As you know, the brain is very hungry and it consumes a lot of energy every day, it cannot work on fats directly, but it can only work on glucose or ketones.

How the ketogenic system works in the body?

Through ketogenic nutrition and when replacing the body's primary energy source, glucose, with a fat source, the body at this stage enters a condition called ketosis, in which case the body becomes a machine for burning fat.

So the body consumes energy from fat instead of glucose and insulin extracted from carbohydrates.

At this stage, **fat is burned continuously throughout the day, 24 hours a day, 7 days a week**.

As it is known, every small movement made by the body needs energy and every mental activity requires energy, even when sleeping the body needs energy! In addition, insulin levels become very low.

And it becomes very easy to burn fat from the stock in the body, this thing is very excellent especially for people who have excess fat in the body, or for people who want to lose weight effectively.

Another benefit is that the body is always in a state of concentration and readiness, because the brain has sufficient energy reserves.

It is worth noting that many studies have shown that this keto diet has mental benefits in terms of concentration and mental activity.

Also worth noting when following this diet is the person does not feel hungry! Unlike other diets like low-fat and low-calorie diets.

When does the ketosis stage occur?

Nice question, this stage occurs when the level of glucose and insulin in the body decreases and this occurs as a result of two options:

The first is in the fasting stage: when the amount of carbohydrates decreases naturally and without counting the amount of carbohydrates.

The second is when reducing carbohydrates and increasing fat in the diet: at this point, the body burns fat through ketones in the liver, as we explained earlier.

Summary: A person cannot fast for long periods. When eating the first meal, the body returns to its state, but when the body is deliberately urged to enter the ketosis stage, the body remains at this stage indefinitely.

People who are not advised to follow a ketogenic diet or a low-carb diet:

There are many rumors and misunderstandings about Keto Diet in terms of safety, but it is safe for most people, except that there are situations that require attention and are the following:

People with type 1 diabetes who take insulin.
People with high blood pressure and who take blood pressure medications.
Breastfeeding and pregnant women.

It should be noted that these states can follow keto and are not prevented from this, but they require them to pay great attention to avoid any problems. Therefore it is advised to consult a specialist before doing this.

Benefits of ketones:

- Increased oxygen in the body
- Increases energy
- Supports the brain
- Supports the heart

Most body tissues can act on ketones, but some parts require glucose. However, you still do not need to take glucose. Your body can build glucose when it needs it through a process called sugar induction.

Why should we get into the ketosis situation?

To reduce insulin

Because high insulin levels cause insulin resistance.

Insulin resistance causes the following diseases:

Symptoms before diabetes

- diabetic
- Metabolic syndrome
- high blood pressure
- Fat in the viscera, especially in the liver

More benefits of the keto and intermittent fasting program:

- Reduces fat in the liver
- Improving cognitive performance
- It improves mood
- Lowering blood pressure
- Reducing inflammation
- Improve energy
- Reducing belly fat
- Self-phagocytosis (recycling damaged proteins and microbes)

Notes:

Hunger disappears with intermittent keto and fasting.

Keto and intermittent fasting work best when combined.

Do not eat unless you are hungry.

Self-phagocytosis (autophagy with significant benefits) begins after about 18 hours of fasting.

During the diet do not forget to increase the salt to overcome any symptoms of dizziness or headache, which are normal symptoms.

What is keto flu?

Keto flu may be a group of symptoms that some people experience once they first start their keto diet.

These symptoms, which can appear almost like influenza, are caused by the body adapting to a replacement diet consisting of only a few carbohydrates.

Reducing the intake of carbohydrates forces the body to burn ketones for energy rather than glucose.

Ketones are byproducts of fat breaking down and become the most fuel source when following a ketogenic diet.

Usually, fats are reserved as a secondary fuel source to be used when glucose isn't available.

This conversion to fat burning for ketosis energy is named. It occurs during certain conditions, including starvation and fasting

However, ketosis also can be achieved through a low-carb diet.

In a ketogenic diet, **carbohydrates are usually reduced to but 50 grams per day**

This dramatic decrease can come as a shock to the body and should cause withdrawal-like symptoms, almost like people who occur when weaning from an addictive substance like caffeine

Symptoms

Switching to a low-carb diet may be a big change, and your body may have time to regulate to the present new way of eating.

For some people, this transition period are often especially difficult.

Signs of keto flu may start to seem within the first few days of reducing carbohydrates.

Symptoms can range from mild to extreme and differ between individuals

While some people may switch to a ketogenic diet with none side effects, others may experience one or more of the subsequent symptoms (4 reliable source):

- Nausea
- Vomiting
- Constipation
- Diarrhea
- Headache
- Irritability
- Weakness
- Muscle cramps
- Dizziness
- Weak focus
- Stomach pain
- Muscle soreness
- Difficulty falling asleep
- Sugar cravings

These symptoms are commonly reported by those that have just started a ketogenic diet and may be sad.

Symptoms usually last a few week, although some people may experience them for a extended period of your time.

While these side effects may cause some dieters to throw the towel, there are ways to scale back it.

How to Get obviate the Keto Flu

The keto flu can cause you to feel miserable.

Luckily, there are ways to scale back its flu-like symptoms and help your body get through the transition period more easily.

Stay Hydrated

Drinking enough water with (apple cider vinegar + lemon juices) is important for optimal health and may also help reduce symptoms.

A keto diet can cause you to rapidly shed water stores, increasing the danger of dehydration

This is because glycogen, the stored sort of carbohydrates, binds to water within the body. When dietary carbohydrates are reduced, glycogen levels fall and water from the body is excreted

Staying hydrated can help with symptoms like fatigue and muscle cramping

Replacing fluids is particularly important once you are experiencing keto-flu-associated diarrhea, which may cause additional fluid loss

Avoid Strenuous Exercise

While exercise is important for staying healthy and holding weight in control, stressful exercise during symptoms of keto-flu should be avoided

Fatigue, muscle cramps and stomach discomfort are common within the first week of following a ketogenic diet, so it's going to be an honest idea to offer your body a rest.

Activities like intense biking, running, weight lifting and strenuous workouts may need to be placed on the rear burner while your system adapts to new fuel sources.

If you experience keto flu, these kinds of exercises should be avoided, but light activities such as walking, yoga, or leisurely biking can improve symptoms.

Replace electrolytes

Replacing electrolytes in the diet may help to reduce symptoms of keto-flu..

When following a ketogenic diet, levels of insulin, a crucial hormone that helps the body absorb glucose from the bloodstream, decrease.

If insulin levels decrease, the kidneys release excess sodium from the body. Moreover, the keto diet restricts many potassium-rich foods,

potassium-rich foods	magnesium	phosphorous	calcium	Vitamin B1
Spinach.	Dark Chocolate	Pork	curly kale	Nutritional yeast
tomato sauce	Avocados	Veal	okra	Flax seed
avocado	almonds	Salmon	spinach	asparagus
parsley	cashews	Mackerel	lemon	Acorn squash
coriander	Brazil nuts	Sardines	sardines	eggs
Dill	flax seed	squash seeds	pilchards	Sunflower seeds
Armenian Cucumber	pumpkin seed	Sunflower seeds	poppy	beef
Oysters	chia seeds	Egg	sesame	pistachio
Salmon	salmon	Yogurt, Greek	Chia seeds	tuna
Watermelon	mackerel	Cheese	celery	Mussels
Yogurt	Halibut.	lamb	almonds	Salmon
Papaya fruits	spinach	beef	collard greens	Macadamia
Beet leaves	turnip greens	Chicken	Broccoli rabe	Oysters

Getting adequate amounts of those important nutrients is a superb thing to power through the different period of the diet.

Salting food to taste and including potassium-rich, keto-friendly foods

These foods also are high in magnesium, which can help reduce muscle cramps, sleep issues and headaches

Get Adequate Sleep

Fatigue and irritability are common complaints of individuals who are adapting to a ketogenic diet.

Lack of sleep causes levels of the strain hormone cortisol to rise within the body, which may negatively impact mood and make keto-flu symptoms worse

If you're having a difficult time falling or staying asleep, try one among the subsequent tips:

Reduce caffeine intake: Caffeine may be a stimulant which will negatively impact sleep. If you drink caffeinated beverages, only do so within the morning so your sleep isn't affected

Cut out ambient light: Shut off cell phones, computers and televisions within the bedroom to make a dark environment and promote restful sleep

Take a bath: Adding Epsom salt or lavender volatile oil to your bath may be a relaxing thanks to wind down and obtain ready for sleep

Get up early: Waking at an equivalent time a day and avoiding oversleeping may help normalize your sleep patterns and improve sleep quality over time.

Make Sure you're Eating Enough Fat and vegetables

Transitioning to a really low-carb diet can cause you to crave foods that are restricted on the ketogenic diet, like cookies, bread, pasta and bagels.

However, eating enough fat, the first fuel source on the ketogenic diet, will help reduce cravings and keep you feeling satisfied.

In fact, research shows that low-carb diets help reduce sweet and high-carb diet cravings

Those having a difficult time adapting to the ketogenic diet may need to eliminate carbohydrates gradually, instead of all directly.

Slowly curtailing on carbs, while increasing fat and protein in your diet, may help make the transition smoother and reduce keto-flu symptoms.

Why do some people get Keto flu?

People adapt to ketogenic diets differently. While some people may experience weeks of keto flu symptoms, others may adapt to the new diet with none harmful side effects.

The symptoms people experience are associated with how their bodies adapt to a replacement fuel source.

Usually, carbohydrates provide the body with energy within the sort of glucose.

When carbohydrates are reduced dramatically, the body burns ketones from fat rather than glucose.

Those who consume tons of carbohydrates, especially refined carbohydrates like pasta, sugary cereals and soda, may have a harder time when starting a ketogenic diet.

Thus, switching to a high-fat, low-carb diet could also be a struggle for a few, while others are ready to switch between fuel sources easily with little or no symptoms of the Keto flu.

The reason why some people suits ketogenic diets is simpler than others is unknown, but genetics, loss of electrolyte, dehydration, and carbohydrate withdrawal are believed to be the driving forces behind the keto flu.

How long will it last?

Fortunately, most uncomfortable symptoms of keto flu last a few week for many people.

However, some people may have a harder time adapting to the present high-fat, low-carb diet.

For these individuals, the symptoms may last several weeks.

Fortunately, these symptoms will gradually decrease as your body gets wont to convert ketones into energy.

While symptoms of keto flu are commonly reported by those that switch to a ketogenic diet, if you are feeling a specific malaise and have symptoms like prolonged diarrhea, fever, or vomiting, it's best to contact your doctor to rule out other causes.

How to train on a keto diet?

Many people believe that if you don't consume carbohydrates, you cannot do any exercises so it is not entirely true because your body can actually make sugar through a process called glycation.

So you don't need to eat carbohydrates to get energy too, the energy your body makes (sugar creation) is better and gives you more energy because it is 100% natural from your body also there are other benefits of training while using keto your body makes sugar (glucose formation), and it gets it out through fat Protein, and other enzymes in the body, so it will take you to lose fat faster and get you to your ideal body

How to train?

When you wake up, do some high-intensity cardio exercises before eating any food. Just drink some water, so eat only when you are hungry. Do not eat when you are not hungry because when you do that you stop burning fats because of insulin that tries to reduce blood sugar due to eating

And if you are a heavy lifter, you can also exercise with this type and you are on a diet keto

If you want to increase muscle mass do 8-12 reps

if you want to increase your strength do 1-5 reps

if you want loss fats walk with low intensity about 30-60 min

and the benefits increase when you increase the time but go through it slowly

Food allowed when following a keto diet:

The lower the number of carbohydrates in the nutritional value, the better for entering the ketosis stage, while eating more fat and protein moderately.

The lower the carbohydrate value is less than 6, this means that you will remain in the ideal ketosis stage

Meats that allowed

All kinds of meat are allowed, only the natural source, that is unprocessed and high-fat red and white meats are preferred

Vegetables that allowed

- Spinach
- Lettuce
- Avocado
- Asparagus
- Olives
- Cucumber
- tomato
- Cabbage
- Eggplant
- Zucchini
- Cauliflower
- Kale

- Green beans
- Broccoli
- Pepper green, red, and yellow
- Half carrot
- Half onion
- Half beetroot
- Half rutabaga
- Half celeriac

First, vitamin C, so eat sweet pepper, sauerkraut and lemon.

Secondly omega-3 salmon and greasy are good.

Vitamin B1 III from sunflower seeds and nutritional yeast.

IV iodine is key and obtained seafood and kelp.

 Fifth of iron is also important - get it from red meat or even organ meats (carcass).

Six, phytonutrients from buds and cruciferous are important in hygienic terms and cleaning all chemicals in our environment.

Seven, get potassium and magnesium from 7-10 cups of vegetables.

eat vegetables by 7 to 10 cups per day, and to clarify the amount of cup that he always mentions in his clips we mention an illustrative example with weights of eight cups of fresh vegetables formed in the form of a salad:

A cup of cabbage (crumb) is equivalent to 100 g

Two cups of watercress equivalent to 40 g

A cup of cucumber 120 g

Two cups of lettuce 150 g

Half a cup of tomato 100 g

A cup of fresh mint leaves 25 g

Half a cup of onions 75 g

The total weight is approximately 600g, which is very reasonable for an entire day that you can take in one go or in parts.

Do not forget to add olive oil and lemon and always make sure not to miss the daily amount of vegetables

Fruits are allowed in the keto

- Raspberry: Half a cup (60 grams) contains 3 grams of carbohydrates.
- Black berries: Half a cup (70 grams) contains 4 grams of carbohydrates.
- Strawberry: Eight medium sized grams (100 grams) containing 6 grams of carbohydrates.
- Plum: One medium-sized (65 grams) contains 7 grams of carbohydrates.
- Kiwi: medium grain (70 grams) containing 8 grams of carbohydrates.
- Cherry: Half a cup (75 grams) contains 8 grams of carbohydrates.
- Blueberries: Half a cup (75 grams) contains 9 grams of carbohydrates.
- Clementine: One medium sized (75 grams) contains 9 grams of carbohydrates.
- Melon: One cup (160 grams) contains 11 grams of carbohydrates.
- Peach: One medium-sized (150 grams) contains 13 grams of carbohydrates

Types of oils allowed in keto

- Coconut Oil.
- MCT oil (organic oil made from natural coconut oil powder).
- Extra virgin olive oil.
- Avocado oil.
- butter.
- Animal ghee.
- Liquid cheese (fat).
- Red palm oil.
- Heavy or heavy cream.
- Safflower oil with oleic acid
- Sunflower oil is high with oleic acid

Types of vegetable oils prohibited in the keto diet

1 - soybean oil

This is the most common type of oil, because it is cheap.

It is found in fast-food ingredients, baked goods, French fries, salad dressings, and other foods. The source of soybean oil is genetically modified soybeans.

Linoleic acid also makes up 55% of it, thus contributing to obesity, infections and all the damage we mentioned earlier on linoleic acid.

In addition, it is a well sterilized oil and therefore it is free of any nutritional value, so we advise you to avoid using it.

2 - Peanut oil

Peanut oil is a widely used oil for frying, due to the distinctive flavor it adds to fried food.

However, it is rich in linoleic acid, so its use increases the risk of heart disease, diabetes, cancer and liver disease, and despite its rich content of vitamin E, the damage it causes covers this benefit.

It is better for you to get vitamin E from olive oil and avocado instead of using peanut oil.

3 - corn oil:

It contains a high content of phytocerol, which is vegetable cholesterol, which prevents cholesterol absorption in the intestine, which makes it a reason to lower cholesterol in the body.

This reduces the levels of total cholesterol in the body as well as LDL, but on the other hand, phytoserol has another major harm.

As its height is associated with an increased risk of heart disease in postmenopausal women, and its rise leads to coronary artery problems in men, which increases vascular problems and the risk of heart disease as well.

It may also cause heart disease at a young age, as corn oil is considered the worst among vegetable oils in cooking, because its linoleic acid content is 57%.

4 - canola oil:

All vegetable oils are harmful, but canola oil is not the worst of them. However, it does contain linoleic acid but with less oil

Corn oil and soybeans a lot.

The Food and Drug Administration has agreed to use it to reduce heart disease, mostly due to the high percentage of monounsaturated fatty acids in it which reduces the level of cholesterol in canola oil but reduces cholesterol in the same way in corn oil that uses phytosylate, currently known to be molecules Bad increases the risk of heart disease.

It also contains Erosic Acid, which weakens the ability of the heart and liver to function, so it is best to avoid using this oil in cooking as well.

5 - cottonseed oil:

Cotton does not belong to vegetables, but because the oil is extracted from its seeds and is a plant, so it is considered vegetable oil.

This oil is mainly used in some food brands like Crisco, which many restaurants that need high temperatures rely on to prepare their own meals.

Also, without flavor, it does not affect food, but this oil contains 55% of linoleic acid, which means that these meals served in restaurants cause the entry of large amounts of oxidized fats that are harmful to heart health.

6 - sunflower oil:

Ironically, many brands refer to it as a healthy body oil, because sunflower oil is one of the worst

Vegetable oil.

Contains 60% of linoleic acid.

Additionally, a study was conducted in mice that consumed rich sunflower oil and olive oil, and found very harmful results in the DNA of the group that consumed sunflower oil in their diet.

It increases body aging, disease and cancer, so it is best to avoid it.

7 - safflower seed oil:

This oil is considered the worst ever among vegetable oils, as it contains 70% linoleic acid associated with all the problems we mentioned earlier.

It is also unstable at high temperatures, which leads to its oxidation, which increases the risk of infections and heart diseases, in addition to being free of any nutrients beneficial to the body.

Now that we know what are the worst vegetable oils we should avoid, let us know together the best healthy fat substitutes for these oils.

Keto nuts

Here is our list of the top 7 keto nuts, sorted by carbohydrates.

Pecan Nut - 100 g (3.5 oz) contains 4 g of pure carbs.

Brazilian Nuts - 100gm contains 4gm of pure carbs.

Macadamia - 100 grams contains 5 grams of pure carbohydrates.

Walnuts - 100 grams contain 7 grams of pure carbs.

Hazelnut - 100 gm contains 7 grams of net carbs.

Peanuts - 100 grams contains 8 grams of net carbs.

Almonds - 100 grams contains 9 grams of pure carbs. It can also be ground into almond flour. The neutral flavor makes it a good substitute for high-carb flour, and almond flour can be used in many keto recipes for baking or even pizza.

The best sugar substitutes for keto

If eating sweets helps you eat sweets from time to time, here are the 3 best options:

- Stevia
- Erythritol
- Monk fruit

1. Stevia

Stevia is derived from the leaves of the Stevia rebaudiana plant in South America which belongs to the sunflower family..
Commercial use and marketing of natural leaves is not permitted in the United States. The sweet active compounds, called stevia glycosides, are extracted and purified in a multi-step industrial process to meet American and European regulatory requirements. Although the US Food and Drug Administration did not approve the unrefined papers, it identified the recycled extract as "generally recognized as safe (GRAS)".
Positives
It has no calories and no carbohydrates.

It does not increase blood sugar or insulin levels Seems healthy with low toxicity potential. Stevia is really sweet and goes a little far .
Negatives
Although intensely sweet, it doesn't taste like sugar, and many people find it has a bitter aftertaste.
Food is difficult to cook for results similar to sugar and cannot simply be replaced with existing recipes.
There are not enough long-term data on stevia to distinguish its true effect on the health of frequent users
Sweetness: 200-350 times sweeter than table sugar.
Products: Stevia can be purchased as liquid, powder or granules. Note that granulated stevia products, such as stevia in raw, contain grape sugar. Others, such as Truvia, include erythritol and fillers, and check the ingredient label for all Stevia products.

2. Erythritol

Made from fermented corn or corn starch, erythritol is a sugar alcohol that occurs naturally in small amounts in fruits and fungi such as grapes, melons, and mushrooms.
It is only partially absorbed and digested through the intestine. Erythritol is generally recognized to be safe by the U.S. Food and Drug Administration.
Positives
It contains a small amount of calories and carbohydrates
It does not elevate blood sugar or insulin levels. The active compound goes into the urine without the body needing to use it
In its granular form, it is easy to use to replace real sugar in recipes.
It may prevent dental plaque and dental cavities compared to other sweeteners
Negatives
It doesn't have the same mouth feel as sugar - it has a cold sensation on the tongue.
It can cause bloating, gas, and diarrhea in some people (although not like many other sugar alcohols).
Erythritol absorption and excretion through the kidneys can have negative health consequences (none of them are known at the moment).
We use erythritol in many of our keto candy recipes because it works well in bread and most people tolerate it well.
Sweetness: about 70% as sweet as table sugar.
Products: granulated or powdered erythritol, and stevia mixture. Read ingredient labels to check for dextrose, maltodextrin, or any other additives

3. Monk fruit

Monk fruit is a relatively new alternative to sugar. Also called luo han guo, monk fruit is generally dried and used in herbal tea, soup and broth in Asian medicine. It was cultivated by monks in northern Thailand and southern China, hence its most popular name.

Although fruits in their full form contain fructose and sucrose, the extreme sweetness of the monk fruit is provided by non-caloric compounds called mogrosides, which can replace sugar. In 1995, Procter & Gamble patented a method for extracting solvents from mogrosides from monk fruit.

The US Food and Drug Administration has ruled that monk fruit is generally considered safe. It has not yet been accepted for sale by the European Union, but is expected to be approved in late 2020 or early 2021.

Positives

It does not raise blood sugar levels or insulin.

She has a better taste than Stevia. In fact, it is often mixed with stevia to reduce cost and the weak taste of stevia.

It is also mixed with erythritol to reduce costs and improve cooking use.

It does not cause digestive disorder.

It is very sweet, so a little goes a long way.

Negatives

It's too expensive.

It is often mixed with other "fillers" like insulin, prebiotic fibers and other unstated components.

Be careful with stickers that say "convenience mix", as the product may contain very little monk fruit extract.

Sweetness: 150-200 times as much as sugar.

Products: mix granules with erythritol or stevia, pure liquid drops, or liquid drops with stevia; It is also used to replace products such as sweetened maple syrup from Monk Fruit and chocolate syrup.

Below is a full list of other sweeteners with information on their health and safety profiles, and whether they are safe for keto

Sugar alcohol

Sugar, also known as polyols, tastes sweet but does not contain alcohol (ethanol). Its effects on blood sugar and insulin levels vary according to the type used. The sugar alcohol mentioned below is generally recognized as safe (GRAS) by the American FDA.

Alcoholic drinks that allowed in the keto diet?

First, it is clear: Alcohol does not help in losing weight. The more alcohol you drink, the more difficult it will be to lose weight, because the body tends to burn alcohol before anything else. Drinking alcohol can also make you want to eat more.

There is a big difference between the different types of drinks when it comes to the number of carbohydrates they contain. Some are fine, others are disasters.

Short version: Wine is much less carbohydrate than beer, so most people choose keto wine.

Pure spiritual drinks such as whiskey and vodka contain zero carbs. Watch out for sweet mixed drinks - they may contain large amounts of sugar.

dry white wine

Weiss says different types like sauvignon blanc, Italian pinot grigio, and pinot blanc are low-carb options. "All of these contain about 1 gram of carbohydrates per ounce, or less," she says. For example, one cup of 5 ounces of sovignon planet contains 3 grams of carbohydrates, 0 grams of fat and 0.1 grams of protein, according to the USDA.

Dry red wine

Weiss recommends Cabernet Sauvignon, Pinot Noir or Merlot cells, which are drier varieties that provide less carbohydrates per ounce of sweet red wine. One cup of cabernet sauvignon contains 3.8 grams of carbohydrates, 0 grams of fat and 0.1 grams of protein. If you are looking for a great brand, she loves Dry Farm Wines, a wine club that offers small sugar-free farms and low-alcohol wines.

Champagne or Prosecco

Start emptying bottles (responsibly). Champagne gets a green light from Weiss because it will contain less than 1g of carbs per ounce. Look for protein (instead of "extra dry" or "sweet") that contains less carbohydrates. A standard 5-ounce cup of California Champagne called Korbel contains 4g of carbs, 0g of fat and 0g of protein.

Hard Liquor

"Lives do not contain carbohydrates," says Olivia Wagner, RDN, an integrated nutritionist. Drink 1 ounce of your favorite hard liquor - vodka, tequila, rum, gin, or whiskey - and add a mixer like soda water or sparkling flavored water (like LaCroix or Waterloo) to a drink without calories, sugar, or carbohydrates. For reference, a single tequila dose contains 0g of carbohydrates, fats and protein for 97 calories. Note that alcohol contains 7 calories per gram.

Mojito

The standard mojito - made with rum, lemon juice, mint, sugar and soda water - contains just 5g of pure carbs (plus 0g of fat and 0.2g of protein). This will make up a lot of carbohydrates on that day, but it can be contained on a day when you want a mixed drink. But you can do better with a twist on the mojito, says Wagner. Get rid of sugar, add rum to roast mint, soda water, and cover lime.

The worst alcohol choices on keto diet

Beer

Sorry, but whether you like luxury IPAs, beers, or beers, beer is, if not light, outside. (For example, a 12-ounce Bud Light package contains just 4.6 grams of carbohydrates.) 'Beer is made of barley and then processed into sugar. Then yeast, which works on this sugar, is added to more carbohydrates. With Keeping in mind that a beer can (12 fluid ounces) contains 13 g of carbohydrates, 0 g of fat and 1.7 g of protein, you can get one beer and then you should severely limit the rest of your carbohydrates for the day. It says, "If you were wasting carbohydrates on beer, you couldn't eat green vegetables or berries." All that said, a carbohydrate ration is not a healthy way to use. (Oh, and if you can't live without beer, the keto diet may not be right for you, she says.)

Vodka tonic

Fortified water contains tons of sugar. It's tricky because it is often confused with soda water, and it's only H20 carburetor (i.e. it doesn't contain carbohydrates or calories). On the other hand, vodka tonic contains 15 grams of carbohydrates (all of them added sugar in fortified water), 0 grams of fat, and 0 grams of protein.

Diet coke (or regular coke) and rum

Many people on a keto diet tend to eat artificial sweeteners. Although Keto is friendly, experts usually advise against it. "I have clients who lose weight by removing soft drinks from the diet," says Murray. It goes without saying that soda of any kind - including regular, impermissible soda - is not allowed in keto. A 12-ounce Coca-Cola can contain 39 g of carbohydrates!

Mixed drinks

Most mixed drinks are a mixture of hard wines plus sugar, fruit juice or puree. A few examples? The old fashioned (made with sugar, bitter, and whiskey) contains 10.1 grams of pure carbs, 0.1 grams of fat and 0.3 grams of protein. Margarita contains 36 grams of carbohydrates, 0.2 grams of fat and 0.2 grams of protein.

Mimosa

Yes, it is made from champagne or prosecco, but it also contains a large amount of orange juice, which means a lot of sugar. If you follow a strict keto diet and aim for 20 grams of pure carbs per day, this one drink will eat more than half of your carbohydrate budget. One mimosa contains 12.9 grams of pure carbs, 0.1 grams of fat and less than 1 gram of protein

Typical Keto menu for 14 days

The following list provides but 50 grams of total carbohydrates per day.

As mentioned above, some people may need to reduce carbohydrates further so as to succeed in ketosis.

This is a one-week general keto menu which will be adjusted counting on individual nutritional needs.

Important note:

1. **Drink a small cup of apple cider vinegar and lemon when waking up, before eating and after eating**
2. **Never use sugar (there is a diet sugar called (stevia ... etc.)**
3. **Not to eat rice, pasta, pie, bread, or fruits (fruits after the first week, but certain fruits)**
4. **How to make a lemon and apple cider vinegar drink (a liter of water with 4-5 small spoons of apple cider vinegar and squeeze half of a lemon juice and sweeten it with a teaspoon of stevia)**
5. **Drinking Anise after eating improves digestion.**
6. **vegetables that i mentioned on the schedule :**
     An illustrative example of the required daily amount of vegetables
   - A cup of bell pepper 100 g
   - Two cups of watercress 40 grams
   - A cup of cucumber 120 grams
   - Two cups lettuce 150 grams
   - Half a cup of tomatoes 100 g
   - A cup of fresh mint leaves 25 c
   - Half a cup of onions 75 g
   - Coriander 50g, parsley 50g, dill 50g (if there is no lettuce or watercress)

Saturday:
Meal 1: 2 fried chicken thigh and vegetables, then 50 g of Sunflower seeds
Meal 2: 6 eggs fried with eggplant or as much as you like, and they have motley and vegetables, then 50 grams of Sunflower seeds

❖ Sunday:
Meal 1: large mackerel fish and vegetables
Meal 2: a large fried chicken thigh and vegetables or 6 eggs and vegetables

❖ Monday
Meal 1: 150 g of liver, cut into pieces and cooked with (bell pepper and half a large onion) with butter and two boiled eggs
Meal 2: 6 eggs fried with mozzarella, then 50g of Sunflower seeds

❖ **Tuesday**

The meal 1: 2 natural beef hamburger fried with butter and vegetables
Meal 2: 150 grams of tuna with vegetables, on them 3 tablespoons of olive oil

❖ **Wednesday**

Meal 1: 200 g of meat with fat and vegetables
Meal 2: 6 eggs boiled with butter and vegetables

❖ **Thursday**

Meal 1: large mackerel fish and vegetables
Meal 2: 2 hamburger or 150 g tuna or 6 eggs and vegetables

❖ **Friday**

Meal 1: 200 grams of meat with fat and vegetables
Meal 2: a large fried chicken thigh and vegetables

The most important note is drinking apple cider vinegar and lemon before and after eating and upon waking up

❖ **Monday**

Breakfast: two fried eggs in moistened butter, served with sauteed vegetables.
Lunch: a burger without bread covered with herb topped with cheese, mushrooms and avocado on a layer of vegetables.
Dinner: pork slices or salmon or tuna with green beans in coconut oil.

❖ **Tuesday**

Breakfast: omelette.
Lunch: tuna fish salad with celery and tomato on top of a bed of vegetables.
Dinner: grilled chicken with cream sauce and fried broccoli.

❖ **Wednesday**

Breakfast: sweet pepper full of cheese and eggs.
Lunch: watercress salad with boiled eggs, turkey, avocado and blue cheese.
Dinner: grilled salmon with spinach in coconut oil.

❖ **Thursday**

Breakfast: whole milk topped with Granola Quito.
Lunch: a steak bowl with broccoli rice, cheese, herbs, avocado and sauce.
Dinner: bison steak with cheese broccoli.

❖ **Friday**

Breakfast: baked avocado eggs boats.

Lunch: Caesar salad with chicken.

Dinner: pork chops with vegetables.

❖ Saturday

Breakfast: Cauliflower bread topped with cheese and avocado.

Lunch: salmon burger without bread topped with pesto.

Dinner: served meat balls with zucchini noodles and parmesan cheese.

❖ Sunday

Breakfast: shea pudding with coconut milk with coconut and walnuts.

Lunch: A cup salad made with vegetables, boiled eggs, avocado, cheese and turkey.

Dinner: coconut chicken curry.

Breakfasts

❖ Classic bacon and eggs

Ingredients
8 eggs
150 g bacon, in slices cherry
tomatoes (optional)
fresh parsley (optional)

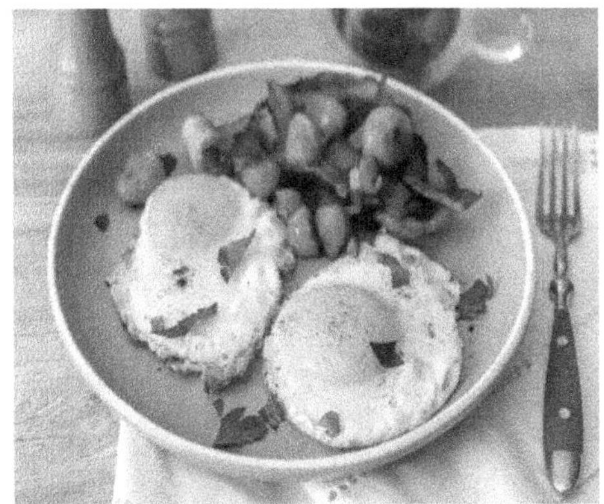

- Instructions

Fry the bacon during a pan on medium high heat until crispy. forgot on a plate. Leave the rendered fat within the pan.

Use an equivalent pan to fry the eggs. Place it over medium heat and crack your eggs into the bacon grease. you'll also crack them into a cup and punctiliously pour into the pan to avoid splattering of hot grease.

Cook the eggs any way you wish them. For sunny side up — leave the eggs to fry on one side and canopy the pan with a lid to form sure they get cooked on top. For eggs cooked over easy —

flip the eggs over after a couple of minutes and cook for an additional minute. Cut the cherry tomatoes in half and fry them at an equivalent time.

Salt and pepper to taste.

Tip!

Step up your bacon game with organic bacon if you'll find it… it's tastier and has fewer additives..

❖ **Boiled eggs with mayonnaise**.

Ingredients
8 eggs
8 tbsp mayonnaise
2 avocados (optional)

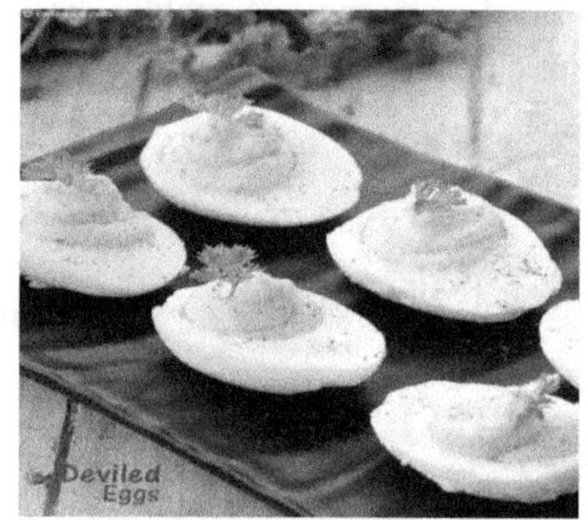

- Instructions

Bring water to a boil during a pot.

Optional: Make tiny wholes within the eggs using an egg piercer. This helps prevent eggs from cracking while boiling.

Carefully, place the eggs within the water.

Boil the eggs for 5–6 minutes for soft-boiled eggs, 6–8 minutes for medium and 8–10 minutes for hard-boiled eggs.

Serve with mayonnaise.

Serving suggestion

Enjoy your eggs with some avocado and/or fried asparagus with homemade mayonnaise. Another super-simple option is to eat the boiled eggs with butter. Mash them together during a small bowl. Add some fresh herbs if you're within the mood. Delicious!

❖ **Keto Mexican scrambled eggs**

Ingredients
30 g butter
1 scallion, finely chopped
2 pickled jalapeños, finely chopped
1 tomato, finely chopped
6 eggs
75 g shredded cheese salt and pepper

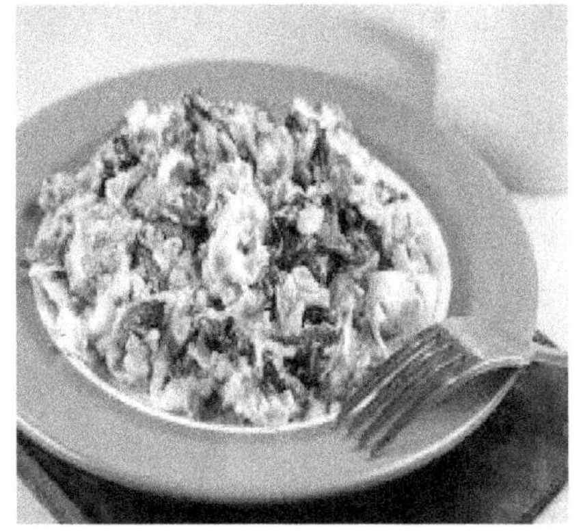

- instructions

Melt butter in a large frying pan over medium-high heat.

Add the scallions, jalapenos and tomatoes and fry for 3-4 minutes.

Beat the eggs and place them in the pan. Scramble for a couple of minutes. Add the cheese and the seasoning..

❖ **Keto avocado eggs with bacon sails**

Ingredients
2 hard-boiled eggs
½ avocado
1 tsp olive oil

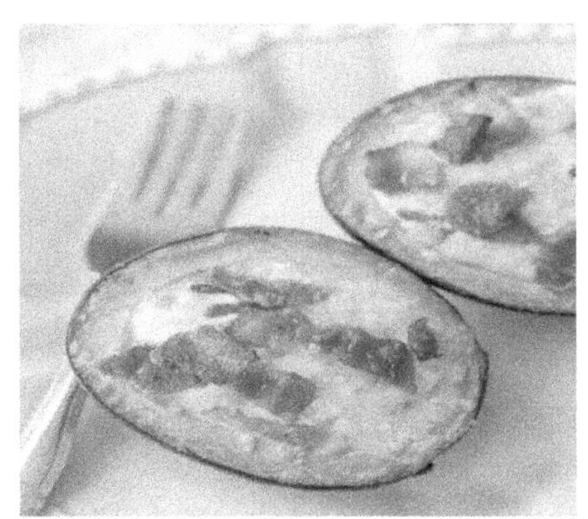

75 g bacon salt and pepper

- instructions

Preheat the oven to 180 ° C (350 ° F).

Put the eggs in a saucepan and cover with water. Bring to a gentle boil and cook for 8-10 minutes. Place the eggs in ice cold water as soon as they are done to make them easier to peel.

Cut the eggs in half lengthwise and scoop out the yolks. Place in a small bowl.

Remove avocado and oil and mix once mixed. Salt and chili pepper to compare.

Put the bacon on a baking sheet and cook until crisp. It's going to take around 5–7 minutes. You may even cook them in a frying pan.

Carefully add the mixture back to the cooked egg whites with a spoon and set the bacon sail! Enjoy it!.

❖ Keto breakfast tapas

Ingredients
110 g cheddar cheese
225 g prosciutto
225 g chorizo
125 ml mayonnaise
110 g cucumber
50 g red bell peppers

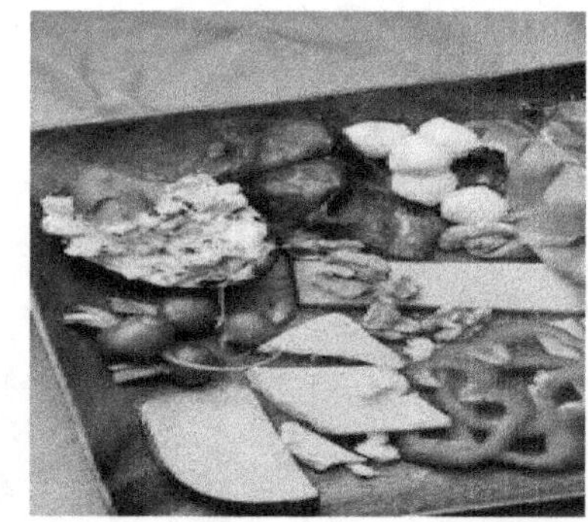

- instructions

Cut the cold cuts, cheeses and vegetables into sticks or cubes.

Arrange it on a plate, serve it and enjoy it.

❖ **Scrambled eggs with basil and butter**

Ingredients
2 tbsp butter
2 eggs
2 tbsp heavy whipping cream salt and ground black pepper
50 g shredded cheese
2 tbsp fresh basil

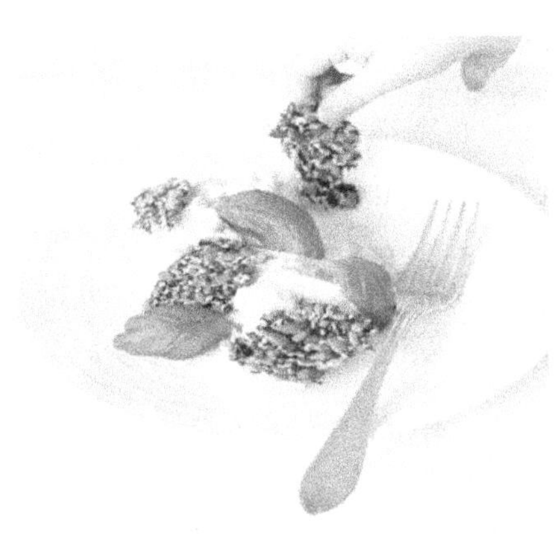

- instructions

Melt the butter in a low heat pan.

In a shallow tub, incorporate cracked eggs, cream , cheese and seasoning. Give it a light whisk and add it to the pan.

Stir the spatula from the edge to the middle before the eggs are scrambled. If you want to be smooth and fluffy, mix on a low heat before consistency is needed.

Cover with a new basil.

Suggestion to serve

Have your scrambled eggs with about 1–1 1/2 oz (30–50 g) butter, lots of fresh herbs and, ideally, a few pieces of low-carb sesame crispbread. Enjoy it!

❖ **Low-carb baked eggs**

Ingredients
75 g ground beef or ground lamb or ground pork, use left-overs or cook it any way you like. You can also use this recipe.
2 eggs
50 g shredded cheese

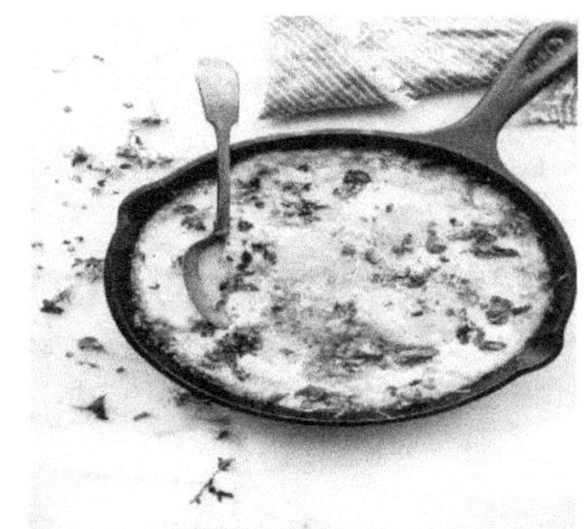

- instructions

Preheat the oven to 200 ° C (400 ° F).

Arrange the ground beef mixture in a tiny baking dish. Then make two holes with a spoon and crack the eggs.

Sprinkle with shredded cheese on top.

Bake in the oven until the eggs have done, around 10-15 minutes.

Let's just cool for a while. Eggs and ground meat are getting very hot.

Tip!

This is the perfect recipe for the leftover burger you weren't quite sure what to do with. Multiply the recipe by the number of people and you're going to have dinner for the whole family. Hey, Voila!

Pair with a crisp, crunchy, green salad of fresh herbs and avocado. Or try this delicious homemade mayonnaise (made without soybean oil and additives).

This is a perfect recipe for that leftover hamburger you weren't quite sure what to do with. Multiply the recipe by the number of people and you'll have dinner for the whole family. Voila!

Pair it with a crisp, crunchy, green salad with fresh herbs and avocado. Or try it with this scrumptious homemade mayonnaise (made without soybean oil and additives).

Meals

❖ **Keto pizza:**

Ingredients
Crust
4 eggs
175 g shredded cheese, preferably mozzarella or provolone Topping
3 tbsp unsweetened tomato sauce
1 tsp dried oregano
150 g shredded cheese
40 g pepperoni olives (optional) For serving
50 g leafy greens
4 tbsp olive oil sea salt and ground black pepper

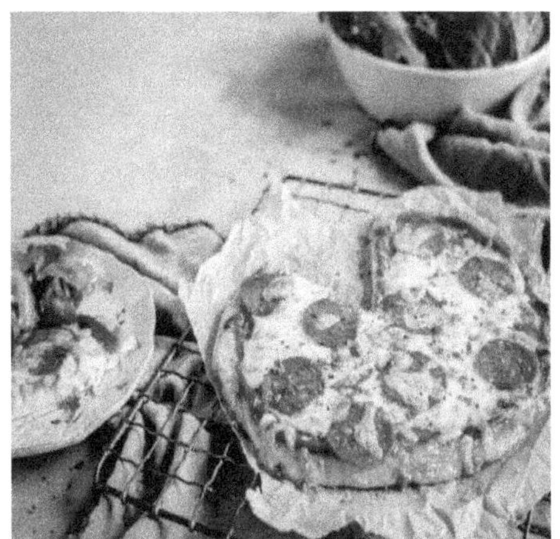

- Instructions

Preheat the oven to 400°F (200°C).

Start by making the crust. Crack eggs into a medium-sized bowl and add shredded cheese. provides it an honest stir to mix.

Use a spatula to spread the cheese and egg batter on a baking sheet lined with parchment paper. you'll form two round circles or simply make one large rectangular pizza. Bake within the oven for quarter-hour until the pizza crust Increase the oven temperature to 450°F (225°C).

Spread tomato sauce on the crust and sprinkle oregano on top. Top with cheese and place the pepperoni and olives on top.

Bake for an additional 5-10 minutes or until the pizza has turned a golden brown color.

Serve with a fresh salad on the side..

❖ **Keto hamburger patties with creamy tomato sauce and fried cabbage:**

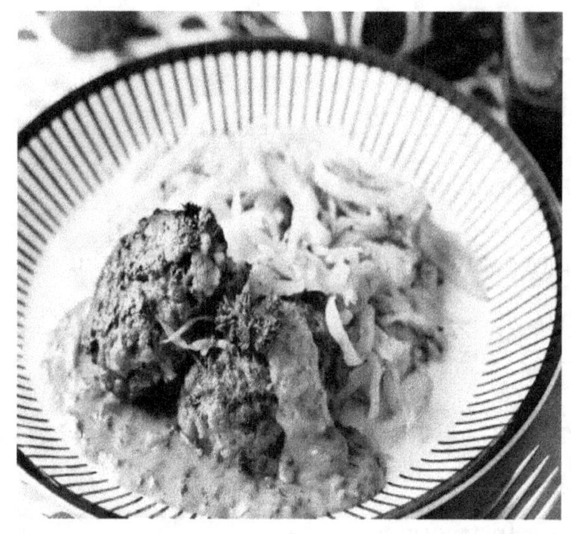

Ingredients
1½ lbs ground beef
1 egg
3 oz. crumbled feta cheese
1 tsp salt
¼ tsp ground black pepper
2 oz. fresh parsley, finely chopped
1 tbsp olive oil, for frying
2 tbsp butter, for frying Gravy
¾ cup heavy whipping cream
1 oz. fresh parsley, coarsely chopped
2 tbsp tomato paste or ajvar relish salt and pepper Fried green cabbage
1½ lbs shredded green cabbage
4½ oz. butter salt and pepper

- Instructions
    - Hamburger patties and gravy

Add all ingredients for the hamburgers to an outsized bowl. Blend it employing a wooden spoon or your clean hands. Don't over mix since which will make your patties tough. Use wet hands to make eight oblong patties.

Add butter and olive oil to an outsized frying pan. Fry over medium-high heat for a minimum of 10 minutes or until the patties have turned a pleasant color. Flip them a couple of times for even cooking.

In a small bowl, whisk together the tomato paste and cream. Add this mixture to the pan when the patties are almost done. Stir and let simmer for a couple of minutes. Salt and pepper to taste.

Sprinkle chopped parsley on top before serving.

-   Butter-fried green cabbage

Shred the cabbage finely employing a food processor or sharp knife.

Add butter to an outsized frypan.

Place the pan over medium high heat and sauté the shredded cabbage for a minimum of quarter-hour or until the cabbage is wilted and golden brown round the edges.

Stir regularly and lower the warmth a touch towards the top. Add salt and pepper to taste.

Tip!

Switch it up! These patties pair well with any sautéed vegetable… What does one love? Onions, mushrooms, spinach, Brussels sprouts, asparagus, green beans……

❖ **Keto BLT with cloud bread:**

Ingredients
3 eggs
4 oz. cream cheese
1 pinch salt
½ tbsp ground psyllium husk powder
½ tsp baking powder
¼ tsp cream of tartar (optional) Filling

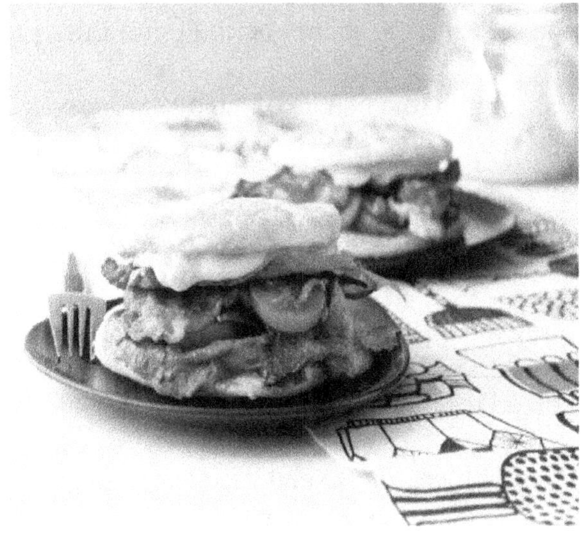

4 tbsp mayonnaise
5 oz. bacon
2 oz. lettuce
1 tomato, thinly sliced

- Instructions
  - Cloud bread

Preheat oven to 300°F (150°C).

Separate the eggs, with egg whites in one bowl and egg yolks in another. Note, egg whites whip better during a metal or ceramic bowl as against plastic.

Whip egg whites along side salt (and cream of tartar, if you're using any) until very stiff, preferably employing a hand-held mixer. you ought to be ready to turn the bowl over without the egg whites moving.

Add cream cheese, psyllium husk and baking powder and mix well.

Gently fold the egg whites into the egg yolk mixture — attempt to keep the air within the egg whites.

Place two dollops of the mixture per serving on a paper-lined baking tray. opened up the circles with a spatula to about ½ inch (1 cm) thick pieces.

Bake within the middle of the oven for about 25 minutes, until they turn golden.

  - Building the BLT

Fry the bacon during a skillet on medium high heat until crispy.

Place the cloud bread pieces top-side down.

Spread mayonnaise on each bread.

Place lettuce, tomato and fried bacon in layers between the bread halves..

❖ **Keto turkey with cream-cheese sauce:**

Ingredients
2 tbsp butter
1½ lbs turkey breast
2 cups crème fraîche or heavy whipping cream
7 oz. cream cheese
1 tbsp tamari soy sauce salt and pepper
1½ oz. small capers

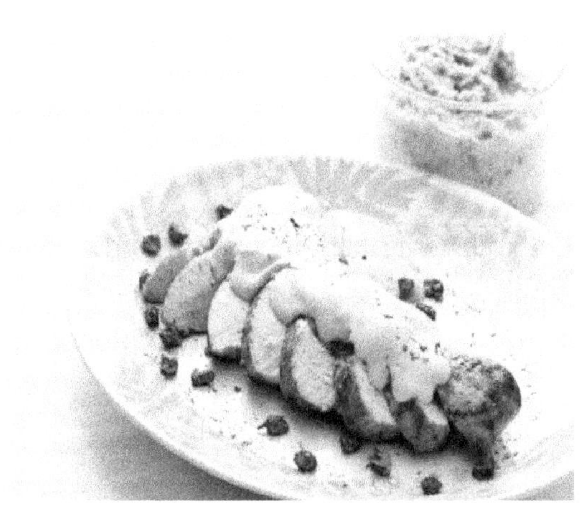

- Instructions

Preheat the oven to 350°F (175°C).

Melt half the butter over medium heat, during a large oven-proof frying pan. Season the turkey generously and fry until golden brown all around.

Finish off the turkey breasts within the oven. When turkey is cooked through and has an indoor temperature of a minimum of 165°F (74°C), place on a plate, and tent with foil.

Pour turkey drippings into alittle saucepan. Add cream and cream cheese. Stir and convey to a light-weight boil. Lower the heat and let simmer until thickened. Add soy, season with salt and pepper.

Heat remaining butter during a medium frypan over high heat. Quickly sauté the capers until crispy.

Serve turkey with sauce and fried capers.

Tip!

Don't forget your side dishes! Both broccoli or cauliflower mash perfectly complement the rich flavors of this turkey. And celebrate with this supremely versatile cream cheese sauce! It are often adapted to any quite boneless or bone-in meat you prefer. Fillets or chops. Beef or pork. Lamb or chicken. Just remember to stay the skin or fat on when possible, as this really enhances flavor and fat content.

Let your imagination be your guide! There are numerous flavor combinations to try: tapenade, pimientos, tomato paste, parmesan cheese, fresh herbs, fried onion, garlic, curry paste, lemon and capers all work beautifully with this recipe..

❖ **Keto oven-baked Brie cheese:**

Ingredients
9 oz. Brie cheese or Camembert cheese
1 garlic clove, minced
1 tbsp fresh rosemary, coarsely chopped
2 oz. pecans or walnuts, coarsely chopped
1 tbsp olive oil salt and pepper

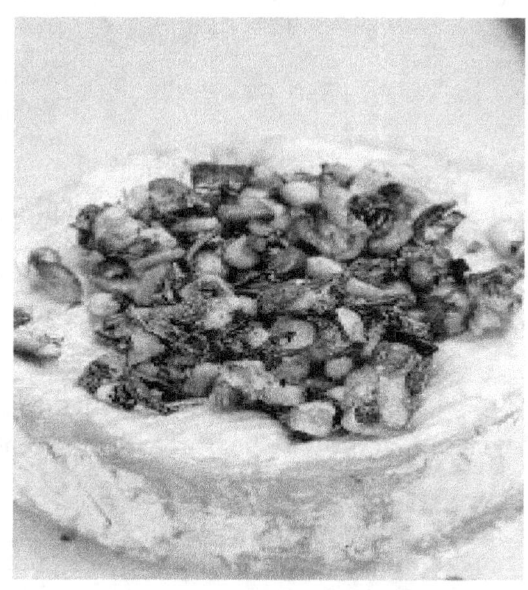

- Instructions

Preheat the oven to 400°F (200°C).

Place the cheese on a sheet pan lined with parchment paper or during a small nonstick baking dish.

In a small bowl, mix the garlic, herb and nuts along side the olive oil. Add salt and pepper to taste.

Place the nut mixture on the cheese and bake for 10 minutes or until cheese is warm and soft and nuts are toasted. Serve warm or lukewarm.

Tip!

If you're feeding a crowd, use a bigger wheel of Brie. Just double or triple the topping ingredients and plan for more baking time. Serve with keto seeded crackers or thinly sliced pears or apples if you'll tolerate fruit. Or alone with a fork.

Mix up the herbs! you'll also use fresh parsley or thyme to urge new exciting flavor combos..

❖ **Keto pimiento cheese meatballs:**

Ingredients
Pimiento cheese
1/3 cup mayonnaise
¼ cup pimientos or pickled jalapeños
1 tsp paprika powder or chili powder
1 tbsp Dijon mustard

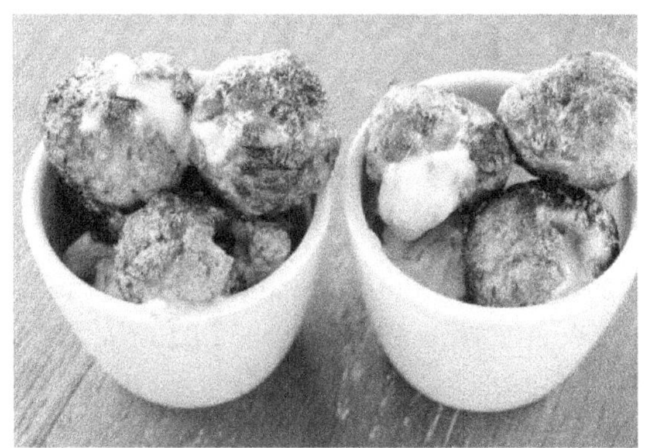

1 pinch cayenne pepper
4 oz. cheddar cheese,
Meatballs
1½ lbs ground beef
1 egg
salt and pepper
2 tbsp butter, for frying

- Instructions

Mix chipotle paste, oil and salt during a small bowl.

Brush the meat with the marinade and let sit for 15 minutes. you'll also marinate the meat during a bag for half-hour or more within the fridge.

Preheat the oven to 400°F (200°C). Grill the marinated meat on a rack on a baking sheet within the oven for 20–30 minutes until the meat is thoroughly done. Turn after 10-15 minutes.

Meanwhile, prepare the garlic butter and therefore the beans. Press the garlic clove, mix with butter and spices and put aside.

Heat the oil during a frying pan. Sauté the beans for about 5 minutes on medium high heat until they need turned a pleasant color. Lower the heat towards the top, and add spices.

Chop the onion finely. Peel and take away the pit from the avocado and mash the flesh coarsely with a fork. Stir onion and avocado into the beans. Season with salt and pepper to taste. Top with a couple of finely chopped cilantro.

Tip!

Grilling meat within the oven is super convenient because it takes care of itself. But, be happy to fry the chops during a frypan or toss them on the grill. Whichever cooking method you favor, you'll still get chipotle deliciousness!!

❖ **Keto chicken with roasted vegetables Tricolore:**

Ingredients
1 lb Brussels sprouts
8 oz. cherry tomatoes
8 oz. mushrooms
1 tsp sea salt
½ tsp ground black pepper
1 tsp dried rosemary
½ cup olive oil Fried chicken
4 chicken breasts
1 oz. butter, for frying
4 oz. herb butter, for serving

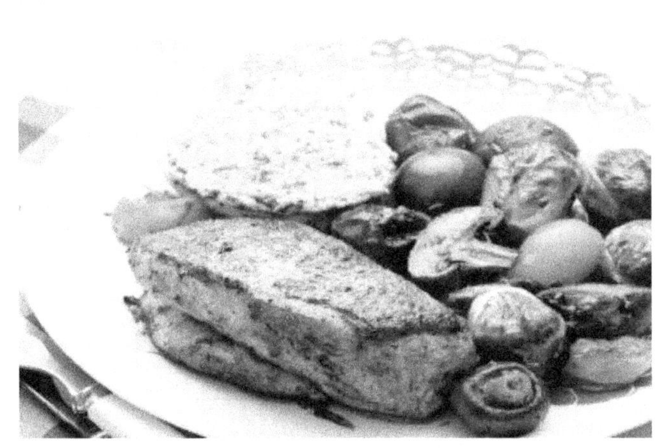

- Instructions

Preheat the oven to 400°F (200°C). Place the vegetables whole during a baking dish.

Add salt, pepper and rosemary. Pour olive oil on top and stir to coat vegetables evenly.

Bake for 20 minutes or until the vegetables are gently caramelized.

Meanwhile, fry the chicken in olive oil or butter and season with salt and pepper. Cook until a thermometer inserted within the largest piece reads 165°F (74°C).

Tip!

Switch up the sauce! This recipe pairs perfectly with a slew of rich sauces. So, don't hesitate to undertake something aside from the herb butter. This healthy and delicious chili aioli may be a fun choice. As are any of those luscious flavored butters..

Bread

❖ **Keto bread**

Ingredients
5 tbsp ground psyllium husk powder
1¼ cups almond flour
2 tsp baking powder
1 tsp sea salt
1 cup water
2 tsp cider vinegar
3 egg whites
2 tbsp sesame seeds (optional)

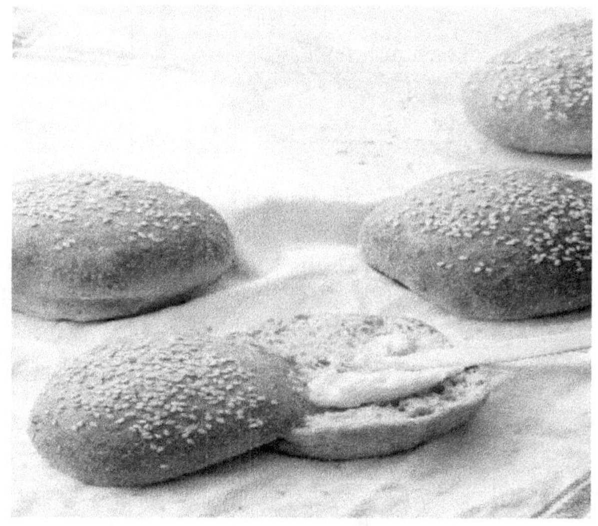

• Instructions

Preheat the oven to 175 ° C (350 ° F).

In a large bowl , mix the dry ingredients. Bring your water to a boil.

Add the vinegar and egg whites to the dry ingredients and mix well. Add boiling water and beat with a hand blender for about 30 seconds. Don't mix the dough over, the consistency should look like Play-Doh.

Moisten your hands with a little olive oil and shape the dough into 6 separate rolls. Put it on a greased baking dish. Top with optional sesame seed.

Bake in the oven on the bottom rack for 50–60 minutes, depending on the size of the bread rolls. They 're finished when you notice a sound as you hit the bottom of the bun.

Serve with the butter and topping of your choice..

❖ **Keto naan bread with melted garlic butter**

Ingredients
175 ml (100 g) coconut flour
2 tbsp (20 g) ground psyllium husk powder
½ tsp onion powder (optional)
½ tsp (2.5 g) baking powder
1 tsp salt 75 ml melted coconut oil
475 ml boiling water coconut oil, for frying (optional) sea salt Garlic butter
110 g butter
2 garlic cloves, minced

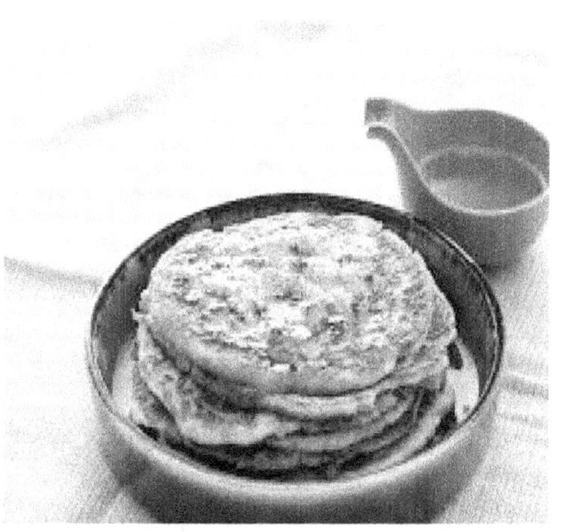

- Instructions

In a pot, mix all the dry ingredients for the keto naan. Add oil and boiling water (hold some of it back if it is not needed) and stir thoroughly.

Allow it to rise for five minutes. The dough is going to be firm very easily, but remain stable. It's expected to imitate the quality of Play-Doh. If you find it too runny, then add more psyllium husk until it feels right. Add some of the remaining water if it's too firm. The quantity you need can differ based on the type of husk or coconut flour you use.

Divide into 6 or 8 parts and turn into balls that you put with your hands directly on parchment paper or on the kitchen counter.Fry rounds in a skillet over medium heat until the naan has a good golden hue. You should apply some coconut oil to it, depending on the pan, so that the bread doesn't stick.

Heat the oven to 70 ° C (140 ° F) and keep the bread warm while making more.

Melt the butter and stir in the freshly pressed garlic. Use a brush to apply the melted butter to the bread pieces and sprinkle the flaked salt on top.

Pour the rest of the garlic butter in a bowl and dip some of the bread in it..

❖ **Soft keto seed bread**

Ingredients
225 ml (110 g) almond flour
175 ml (100 g) coconut flour
75 ml (50 g) sesame seeds
125 ml (100 g) flaxseed
60 ml (40 g) ground psyllium husk powder
3 tsp (15 g) baking powder
1 tsp ground fennel seeds or ground caraway seeds
1 tsp salt
200 g cream cheese, at room temperature
6 eggs
125 ml melted butter or melted coconut oil
175 ml heavy whipping cream
1 tbsp (10 g) poppy seeds or sesame seeds, for topping

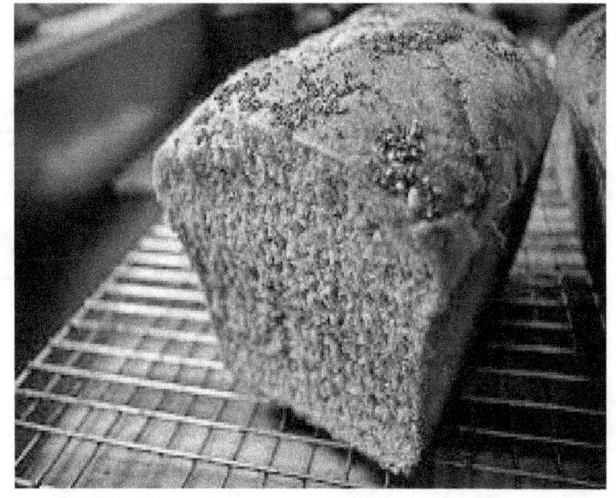

• Instructions

Preheat the oven to 175 ° C (350 ° F).

Mix all the dry ingredients except the topping seeds in a bowl.

In a separate bowl , whisk all remaining ingredients together until smooth.

Add the damp mixture to the dry mixture and mix thoroughly. Place the dough in a greased bread tray, around 4 x 7 inches (non-stick or with parchment paper). Sprinkle over the top with the seeds.

Bake in the oven for about 45 minutes on the bottom rack. Prick the bread with a knife and see if it 's good, it's meant to come out clean. Take it out of the oven and take the bread out of the mold.Remove the paper from the parchment and let the loaf cool down on a rack. Unless the loaf is permitted to cool in the shape of a crust, it may be soggy.

Serve with your favorite toppings, freshly baked.

❖ **Keto coconut-flour bread**

Ingredients
6 eggs
½ cup melted coconut oil
½ cup coconut flour
¼ tsp sea salt
¼ tsp baking powder

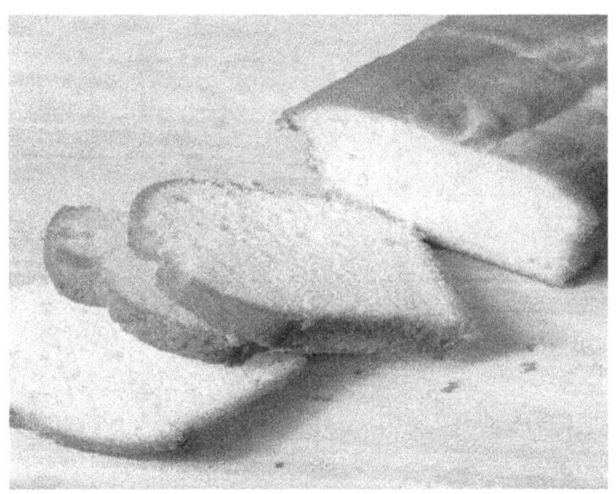

- instructions

Preheat the oven to 175 ° C (350 ° F).

In a large bowl , whisk together eggs and melted coconut oil.

In the same bowl, add the dry ingredients and stir until very smooth.

Grease a small bread pan and fill it with a batter for about 2/3 of the way. Bake for 40-50 minutes or until the toothpick is cold

.Desserts

❖ Old-fashioned keto cake donuts

Ingredients
125 ml (60 g) coconut flour
¼ tsp sea salt
¼ tsp (1.1 g) baking soda
6 eggs 125 ml (100 g) erythritol
125 ml butter or coconut oil
1 tsp vanilla extract
¼ tsp almond extract
Frosting
60 ml melted butter or coconut oil
60 ml cream cheese, softened
60 ml powdered erythritol
½ tsp vanilla extract
Chocolate drizzle
3 tbsp melted butter
2 tbsp powdered erythritol

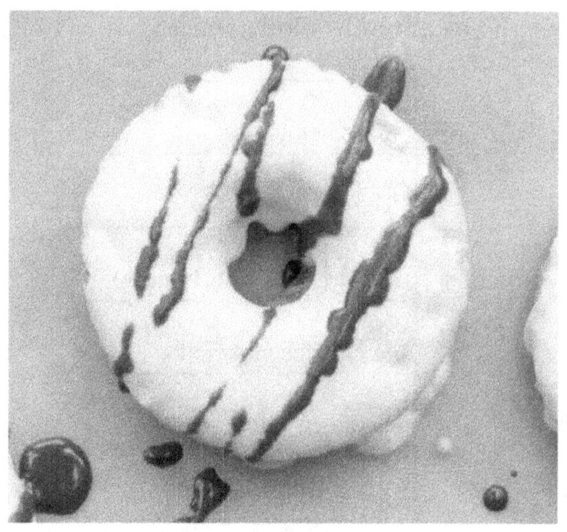

- Instructions

Preheat oven to 350°F (175°C).

In a large bowl, mix the dry donut ingredients together. Stir in the wet ingredients into the dry ingredients. Fill greased donut pan circles about ⅔ of the way full with batter. Bake for about 20 minutes, or until a toothpick comes out clean.

Meanwhile make the frosting by placing all the ingredients in a medium shallow bowl and stir well to combine. Taste and adjust sweetness to your liking.

Dip cooled donuts into the frosting and place on a piece of parchment to chill.

To make the chocolate drizzle, place the ingredients for the chocolate drizzle in a small bowl and stir well to combine. Drizzle donuts with chocolate drizzle if desired.

Tip!

You should make a replacement of tinfoil and a muffin tray if you don't have a donut box. Using a tinfoil square of around 6 "x 6" (15 cm x 15 cm) circle, put a solid central nob in the middle of the foil. Create a donut for rising donut. Click each of them

From the foils to the muffin rings, hold the middle nob and smooth the foil along the edges of each muffin indent. Attach the batter to the foil frame.

You should swap 1⁄2 cup of coconut flour with 2 cups of white almond flour. When you use almond meal, using 2 eggs instead of 6 eggs.

❖ **Kristie's keto carrot cake cheesecake**

ingredients		
Cake batter	Cheesecake filling	Icing
1 tsp apple cider vinegar	16 oz. cream cheese, room temperature	8 oz. cream cheese, room temperature
½ cup heavy whipping cream	2 large eggs	¼ cup unsalted butter, softened
2/3 cup unsalted butter, softened	½ cup erythritol	¼ cup powdered erythritol
1½ cups granulated erythritol	4 drops liquid sweetener	½ tsp vanilla extractInstructions
3 large eggs	1 tbsp vanilla extract	
2 tsp vanilla extract		
2 cups blanched almond flour		
6 tbsp whey protein isolate		
1 tsp ground cinnamon		
¾ tsp baking powder		
½ tsp baking soda		
¼ tsp salt		
½ cup finely shredded carrots		
½ cup walnuts (optional)		

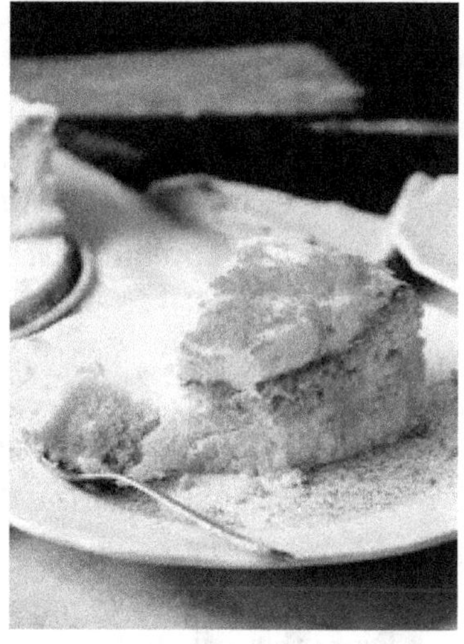

Cake batter

Preheat the oven to 300°F (150°C). Grease a 9-inch (23 cm) springform pan with butter or coconut oil and line with parchment paper.

In a small bowl, mix the vinegar into the heavy whipping cream and set aside.

In a separate bowl, using a hand mixer or stand mixer, cream the butter and granulated sweetener. When the butter has lightened in color, add the eggs one at a time, beating well after each addition. Mix in the vanilla extract and set aside.

In a third bowl, whisk together the almond flour, protein isolate, cinnamon, baking powder, baking soda and salt.

Add the flour mixture to the egg mixture and stir to combine. Stir in the cream mixture. Add the carrots and walnuts, if using, and stir in by hand. The batter will be thick.

Pour the batter into the prepared pan. Use the back of a spoon to push the batter against the sides of the pan, creating a well for the cheesecake filling. Set aside.

Cheesecake filling

In a large bowl, use the mixer to blend the cream cheese, eggs, sweeteners and vanilla extract until smooth.

Carefully pour the filling on top of the prepared cake batter, adding a little filling at a time. Spoon the filling around the center and out and at least ½ inch (1 cm) up the sides of the pan.

Bake for 1 hour 15 minutes to 1 hour 25 minutes, until the edges are browned and the center is set. When the center is set, turn off the oven, leave the oven door slightly open, and let cool for at least an hour. Remove from the oven and let cool completely. Refrigerate for at least 6 hours or overnight.

Cake icing

In a large bowl, use a hand mixer or stand mixer to fully mix all the icing ingredients. Top the cake with the icing. Garnish with a sprinkle of chopped, walnuts or a few shavings of fresh carrot if desired.

Keep in mind!

Also note that while it is great to have a treat or a meal on occasion, it is important to do it just on specific days and not as a regular event. Also, big desserts like this are better eaten as a meal consumed with many, so that you can have one portion, while the other is exchanged with mates and not left as a challenge. This dessert can also be sliced and frozen as an individual serving to avoid overeating.

Tip!

Don't be tempted to double the cake and make a carrot cake layer of cake. The cheesecake crust is the lowest carbohydrate sheet, and the cake is the strongest carbohydrate. Doubling the cake section renders the snack even bigger than the carb

❖ **Keto waffles with blueberry butter.**

Ingredients
150 g melted butter
8 eggs
1 tsp vanilla extract
2 tsp (10 g) baking powder
75 ml (40 g) coconut flour
75 g butter
30 g fresh blueberries

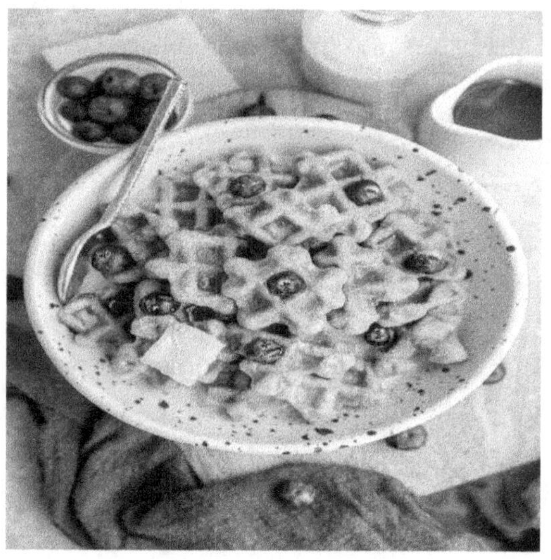

- Instructions

Place the oil and the eggs together. Add the remaining ingredients and combine in a thick mixture using an automatic hand blender.

Allow to rest for 5 minutes and heat the waffle iron to medium.

Upon being adequately baked, dump the batter in the iron and bake until golden. Baking time depends on the thickness of the waffle iron; we packed ours with a 3⁄4 cup (1 1⁄2 dl) flour. Repeat the remaining batter.

Mix butter and blueberries with an electric hand blender and serve with waffles.

Tip!

You don't have time to whip up blueberry butter? Then why not deliver the butter and cinnamon waffles?

❖ **Keto no-bake chocolate cake**

Ingredients
300 ml heavy whipping cream or coconut cream
3 tbsp (35 g) erythritol
200 g sugar-free dark chocolate, stevia sweetened
7 tbsp butter 1 pinch sea salt
200 g hazelnuts
100 g (175 ml) pumpkin seeds

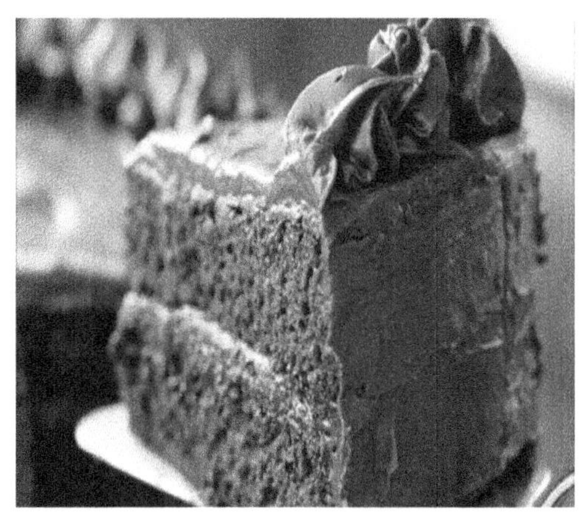

- Instructions

Take heavy cream and sweetener to a simmer in a saucepan. Let it cook for a few minutes before fluffy. Switch the heat off.

Cut chocolate and butter in small pieces and add salt to the hot cream. Stir until chocolate and butter are completely melted and blended.

Roast the hazelnuts and the pumpkin seeds in a large frying pan until crispy and fragrant. Chop it finely and apply nearly half of it to the chocolate and blend. Save some of them for the top.

Place the chocolate mixture in an 8-inch (20 cm) springform pan, preferably covered with parchment paper. Push the parchment paper straight down to protect the base of the plate.Sprinkle with the leftover nuts and seeds, and a sprinkle of sea salt.

Cover with plastic film and put in the refrigerator for about an hour or until the chocolate has hardened

❖ **Keto lemon ice cream.**

Ingredients
1 lemon, zest and juice
3 eggs
75 ml (50 g) erythritol
425 ml heavy whipping cream
¼ tsp yellow food coloring (optional)

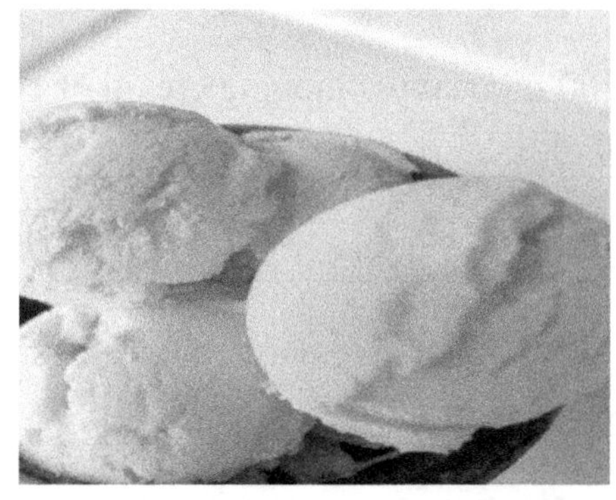

- Instructions

Wash the lemon in warm water. Remove the outer peel (zest) finely. Squeeze the juice out and set aside.

Separate the eggs. Beat the egg whites until they become solid. In another bowl , whisk the egg yolks and the sweetener until light and smooth. Add lemon juice and a few drops of yellow food (optional). Carefully fold the egg whites in the yolk mixture.

Whip the cream in a wide bowl until the soft peaks are created. Add the egg mixture to the cream.

Pour in the ice cream machine and chill according to the manufacturer's directions.

Whether you don't have an ice cream machine, place the bowl in the freezer and mix well every half hour before the perfect consistency is achieved. This might take up to 2 hours.Using a spatula to rub inside the pot when cooking. If frozen, let stand at room temperature 15 minutes before serving.

Tip!

Switch on your citrus! Limes and grapefruit make delicious flavors of ice cream, too. If you try grapefruit, please use one tablespoon of juice for every two servings of ice cream.

❖ **Keto goat cheese with blackberries and roasted pistachios**

Ingredients
550 g goat cheese Blackberry sauce
250 g fresh blackberries
1 tbsp (10 g) erythritol (optional)
1 pinch ground cinnamon Topping
30 g pistachio nuts salt fresh rosemary

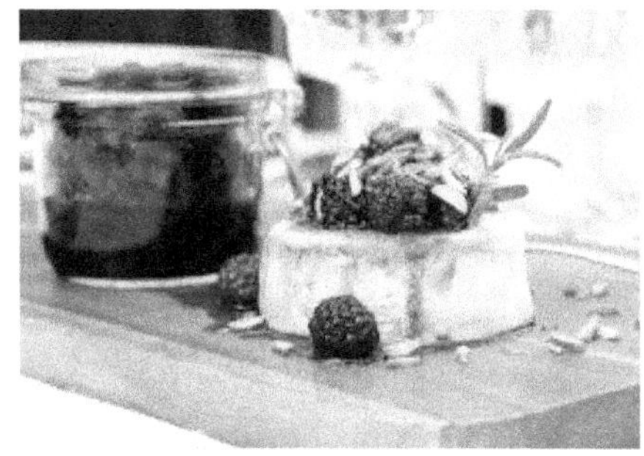

- Instructions

Preheat the oven to 180 ° C (350 ° F).

If used, combine blackberries, cinnamon and sweetener. Place it back.

Bake the goat cheese in the oven for about 10 to 12 minutes or until it has some color. Remove from it and let it rest for a few minutes.

Chop the pistachios and fry them in a dry pan. Adjust to taste with salt.

Finish with blackberry goat cheese, roasted pistachios and rosemary.

Tip!

Blackberries are so delicious and healthy that you do not need any sweeteners, particularly when mixed with cinnamon.

Feel free to swap blackberries with raspberries. If the berries are not juicy enough, microwave them for around 30 seconds. Pistachio is a decent source of protein.Healthy fat and fiber, as well as antioxidants and minerals. Around 50 pistachios have around 5 grams of net carbs and are a very good source of vitamin B6 and potassium. Shelled, raw pistachio can be bought in bulk and is perfect for toasting in this recipe if you don't want to shell your own.

Goat cheese is produced in many varieties and ages. 'Semi-ripened' types, often called soft-ripened goat cheese or semi-ripened goat cheese, are the perfect goat cheese for heating or roasting. It's got a very light rind on the outside and a soft center.

When it's hard to buy semi-ripened goat cheese, you might substitute brie, camembert or other thick rind cheese.

❖ **Keto hard nougat (Turrón)**

Ingredients
175 g macadamia nuts or almonds
225 ml (175 g) erythritol
2 tbsp water
1 large egg white
1 pinch salt

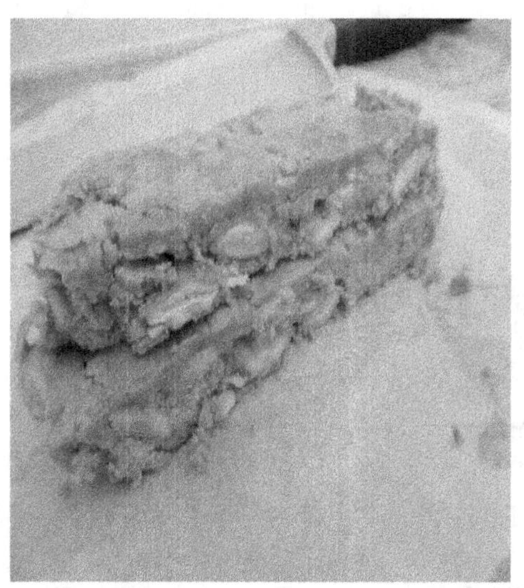

- Instructions

Preheat the oven to 100 ° C (200 ° F).

Line a small pan, approx. 8x6 inches (20 x 15 cm), with parchment paper.

Put the macadamia nuts in a saucepan and cook over medium heat until crispy and toasted. Remove from the heat and add it to the pan.

Combine the erythritol and the water in a small saucepot. Stir occasionally while it heats over medium heat until the mixture is completely fluid, translucent and simmers for about 20 minutes.

While the syrup comes to a simmer, quickly beat the egg white and the salt together until it is white and foamy, almost forming soft peaks.

As you start to whisk the ingredients, gradually mix in the sugar until it is completely mixed.Transfer the egg mixture back to the saucepot and keep stirring with the spatula as you heat over low heat until the egg and the syrup mixture is smooth and sticky for about 30 minutes.

Pour this mixture over the macadamia nuts and smooth it out.

Place the loaf pan in the oven for 2 hours. It's going to clear the mixture so that the candy becomes hot.

Once done , remove from the oven and allow to cool to room temperature before unmolding.

Cut or crack into pieces. Place in paper at room temperature in a cold dry spot.

❖ **Keto vanilla ice cream**

Ingredients
2 egg yolks
1½ cups heavy whipping cream
1 tsp vanilla extract
2 tbsp xylitol
2 egg whites

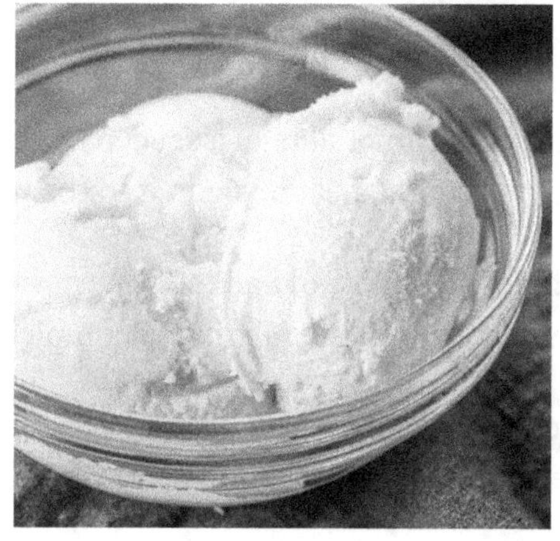

- Instructions

Separate the eggs. Whisk the egg yolks until smooth and fluffy. put aside the egg whites. In a saucepan, combine the cream with the vanilla and therefore the sweetener. bring back a boil and simmer for a couple of minutes, until the cream thickens slightly. Reduce the heat and pour the whipped egg yolks into the recent cream. Combine well and let it simmer on low heat while stirring constantly until the mixture thickens. Refrigerate mixture until cool. Beat the egg whites until stiff and fluffy; fold into the cream mixture. Pour the batter into an ice cream maker or during a jar with a lid and place within the freezer. Stir occasionally and continue freezing until it reaches desired consistency.

Now you can live the ketogenic diet

as a lifestyle without feeling any of

changes in your life

have a good day

by : dr_Loai abdelhamed